SECRETS OF FAITH

CATAMENIAL SOLUTIONS

BY

GLYNIS D. WALLACE D.M.D.

All Rights Reserved. No part of this publication may be reproduced in any form or by any means, including scanning, photocopying, or otherwise without prior written permission of the copyright holder. **Copyright © 2016**

DEDICATION

I dedicate this book to my Grandmother ± and Mother ± for instilling a foundation of spiritual connection as the primary mission of achievement, on our journey through life. To my husband who is always standing by my side much thanks and gratitude

Acknowledgements

To all who realize the government funds science, so it is progressing rapidly, and we must expose all willing to listen to alternative energy like Faith and its gifts to sustain life.

"If you want to find the secrets of the universe, think in terms of energy, frequency, and vibration."

— *Nikola Tesla*

"Energy has no beginning and no end."

— *Nikola Tesla*

CONTENTS

Introduction

Chapter 1 1

Spiritual foundation

Chapter 2 3

What is Faith

CHAPTER 3 5

Trials That Increased My Faith

CHAPTER 4 13

Medicinal Gifts from the Bible

CHAPTER 5 25

Breath of Life

Chapter 6 28

Mission and Purpose

Revealed in a Dream

INTRODUCTION

In your greatest time of need, there can be comforting energy that engulfs you from a higher power. This power is extraordinary intense unnatural or supernatural. I have been privileged to experience this energy force at times when FEAR tends to stand for forgetting everything's all right. Many trials occurred to break my spirit and challenge my beliefs. Uncertainty and turmoil of over imagining the worst, but praying and holding on to faith for the best, outcome, revealed a relationship with the mighty universal energy force that words cannot describe. Jesus used the power of faith and worked miracles. This energy is healing and there for all, guiding you to solutions that work. The gifts in this book include the enemies of inflammation to rid you of pain, cancer cures and life preservation herbs in the Bible which changed my life.

Chapter 1
Spiritual Foundation

I was born into a family who believed in prayer, faith and a close walk with God as we journey through life. Sickness overwhelmed my small body at birth, and I was not expected to live. My mother, grandmother and aunties often told me the story of being sent home from the hospital with an undiagnosed illness that the doctors found idiopathic and gave up. Pastor Alexander, the founder of Alexander temple in Texas, looked at my tiny, frail little body and gave me last rights. But as he reached the door, the extraordinary energy (holy spirit) engulfed him, and he grabbed me and held me high praying God would leave me here to be a help unto the nations.

Faith from my mother and the pastor resulted in generous grace for me. They tell me I was extremely pale and lifeless with white stools. A sign of severe anemia which I have experienced my entire life with lung and colon endometriosis: catamenial pneumothorax. Was this the first indication of an issue of blood?

My mother was told by the hospital if I survived the night, to bring me back, so the return trip to the hospital was quite remarkable and surprised many people. Things were very different in those days. Diagnosed with an intolerance to lactose, the sugar in milk, otherwise a healthy infant and placed on a diet of goat's milk, and released. The life force through faith and prayer restored. My health issues through childhood were insignificant.

Who would have imagined the endometrial cells that lined the area which kept me safe for nine months allowing me to grow and develop inside my mother's belly, were now moving through my body wreaking havoc? Just waiting to become Catamenial.

CHAPTER 2
WHAT IS FAITH

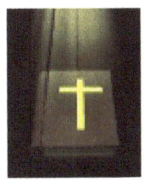

Faith is the exchange module in heaven.

Faith is the foundation of all miracles and mysteries that cannot be analyzed or explained by science.

Faith combined with prayer is a potent unstoppable elixir.

Faith is the remedy to undesirable outcomes.

Faith and prayer give you direct communication with God.

Faith is the foundation that will allow you to rise to your full potential.

Behind your faith, there must be work. "Faith Without Works Is Dead" -James 2:14-26 King James Version (KJV)

Ask for wisdom if you are not sure what work you must accomplish. Wisdom is a gift from God, and through faith, our wisdom matures

Feed your faith and starve your doubts.

Fear has knocked on my door many times, and faith has answered it.

Fear can keep you up all night long, but faith is a pillow of rest.

Faith is standing in the fact that God does not make mistakes, and he designed you for his purpose.

When you pray, if God answers "Yes" he is increasing your Faith, if he responds "Wait" he is increasing your patience. If the answer is "No" he has something better for you!

CHAPTER 3
TRIALS THAT INCREASED MY FAITH

    I was very healthy growing up, hospitalized once at age eleven for a bruised kidney after falling off my bike. I never strayed too far from my spiritual upbringing, but as I began to enjoy life sometimes, I drifted away. There was always a gentle guiding energy force that seems to nudge me back to the familiar life path. My first near death experience in my 30's, was unnerving although enlightening, creating a significant change in my life. I had a new normal, but I did not get my real mission and purpose in life from the experience or at least I did not recognize it. It was confusing, and paranormal experiences began to occur. My actual life mission revealed much later. Maybe that was the reason I had so many recurrent lung collapses without dying. The mission revelation was spectacular. More about that later.

THE BRIGHT LIGHT

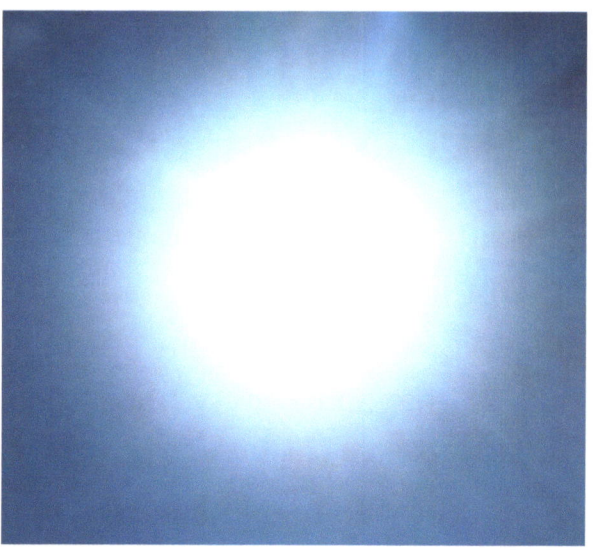

When I entered the Air Force hospital in 1991, it was because of fluid found in my abdomen during an ultrasound. A chest x-ray revealed 3400cc's of blood on my right lung, and removing the fluid led to an introduction to the bright light talked about in near death experiences. The bright light is beautiful, almost bluish white. My legs are limp; my gold shoes fall off, and I can no longer speak with my mouth, but I am talking somehow although it seems they cannot hear me. The light is getting brighter, and I instinctively know I will make it into heaven if I depart the world today.

My eyes are transfixed on the light when I am rudely interrupted as my physician, and medical students began to rush around frantically and remove the tube from my back. I heard them say; we don't want them to mention this in M&M rounds. We were in a room down the hall, but all of a sudden quick movement from the room where I saw the bright light back to my hospital bed.

My mother moves beside me and says her vital signs are 70/40 as the doctor walks toward the door, so does she and I hear her say she's going into shock, he replies I'm so sorry; I hope we can get her back. I never left the bed, but I could see him talking to my mother at the door.

Waking up or coming back to find a full team of doctors 5-10 standing around me. I appeared as if someone had thrown a bucket of water on me. They told me I was being moved to another floor, agreeing as if I had a choice and telling them how tired I felt.

Awakening in the middle of the night, I found someone leaning over me asking if I knew what happened to me. Without hesitation my faith soared, I explained I went into shock, but I am coming all the way back.

Later the nurses asked me if I saw a tunnel with my bright light or people who had passed on. Healthcare workers, who deal with death, seem to know there is a parallel universe. The spiritual world because it is unknown can be frightening. My first Catamenial miracle of survival was evident. The next miracle came one week later with the diagnosis. I called my grandmother and told her I was in trouble, and I needed her to gather the prayer warriors too fast and pray for me. Her answer was unique; she said: "my heart is heavy." They prayed the cells causing fluid in my chest and abdomen was not cancer, tapped into the powerful energy force, holding back a 99% cancer risk and surfacing to the forefront a 1% chance diagnosis of endometriosis. Prayer changed the outcome, a true miracle of faith

I left the hospital a few weeks later and found out my grandmother had asked God for something else. She told God if he needed another soldier in heaven, to take her and leave me here to be a help to the nation. There it was again! I returned from the hospital on Monday, and she went to heaven on Thursday. She told one of my cousins on Sunday; she was going home Thursday, somehow supernaturally, she knew.

A Help to the Nation

I served my country in the United States Public Health Service, later transitioning to the United States Air Force because they were government organizations and it was my way of being a help to the nation. That was not what God had in mind, and of course, he has dreams much bigger for us than we have for ourselves.

After three major surgeries and seven chest tubes, I left active duty military service and found my real purpose. I had a well-documented case of menstrual lung collapse, (Catamenial Pneumothorax) in the world, so I wrote a book to enlighten the nation. Although there were some articles on the subject, "Living With Lung and Colon Endometriosis: Catamenial Pneumothorax" turned out to be the first known book in the world. Many had never heard of it, and now undetermined numbers of women have been diagnosed globally, and it has found a place under pneumothorax diagnosis.

I had taken a lot of medication for many years to suppress the estrogen-driven disease until my hysterectomy including ovaries.

Another trial to test my faith revealed, there is no cure for endometriosis, it's linked to increasing the risk of developing other cancers, and I had developed osteoporosis in my back. There were no medications available to treat my Catamenial Pneumothoraces without making my osteoporosis worst. So the only drugs I have taken in the last fourteen years have been from Gods medicine chest.

I turned to prayer and the remarkable gifts revealed made my life better than I could have ever visualized, with no pain, no side effects. A few flare-ups occurred that were handled without medical intervention, although I did go to the hospital. My faith restored, but a different incident occurred the next time my spirit declined, and fear crept in.

This powerful once in a lifetime occurrence gave me my purpose I was driven to share with others. So starting with my close friends and relatives, a healing force became evident which gave me confirmation; it's time to share it with the nation. The remarkable healing gifts from the Bible that can stop lung collapses, cure cancer, infections, restore memory and give you peace of mind changed my life forever.

CHAPTER 4
MEDICINAL GIFTS FROM THE BIBLE

At baby Jesus birth, he was presented with three gifts whose medicinal value is unmatched. Three wise men traveled to a stable in Bethlehem following a star to deliver Frankincense, Myrrh, and Gold to the king of kings. Gold was possibly the golden spice Turmeric, which cost more than gold at that time. Turmeric is the key to alleviating my pain. This golden spice can change the pain experienced in life. Frankincense (Boswellia) researched and confirmed as a cure for many types of cancer. Myrrh (Guggul) is used to treat many chronic diseases and detoxify the body. Another surprise from the Bible my mother mentioned often seems to help me breathe better instantly after consuming it. It is another well-known spice regular used on pizza, one of our favorite foods. This powerful herb called Hyssop is wild oregano.

TURMERIC

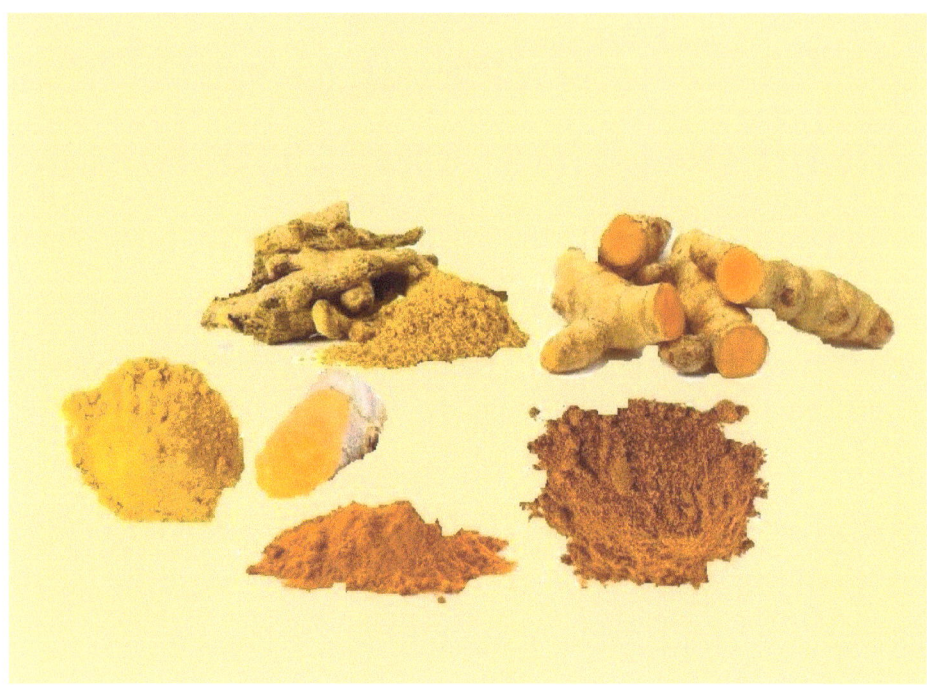

Turmeric is the golden spice with a multitude of uses and is part of my daily diet. It cost more than gold in ancient times and used as a spice as well as a perfume. In India's traditional Ayurveda medicine it was used for whole body healing system. Chinese medicine used it to treat digestive problems, chest congestion, and menstrual discomfort. Curcumin is another name for Turmeric, and in the Bible, it is called Curcuma longa —Song of Solomon 4:14–15

After becoming symptomatic on my left lung in 2006 and fearing a lung collapse on that side, I began to research blocking estrogen naturally. Nature's medicine chest revealed turmeric not only blocked estrogen but a potent anti-inflammatory agent as well. See article "Curcumin inhibits endometriosis endometrial cells by reducing estradiol production" in the reference section." Turmeric is a natural aromatase inhibitor with no side effects and many other health benefits, indeed worth its weight in gold.

In ancient times, Curcumin was used to treat inflammation, flatulence, arthritis, bronchitis, dyspepsia, laryngitis, lymphoma, rheumatism, used as a diuretic and expectorant.

Turmeric (Curcumin) is anti-tumor, inhibiting cancer growth, and protects healthy cells from radiation and chemicals.

Finding this superb healing spice gave me piece of mind, so I put it in the water when cooking rice or noodles and season all of my meats and vegetables with it.

FRANKINCENSE

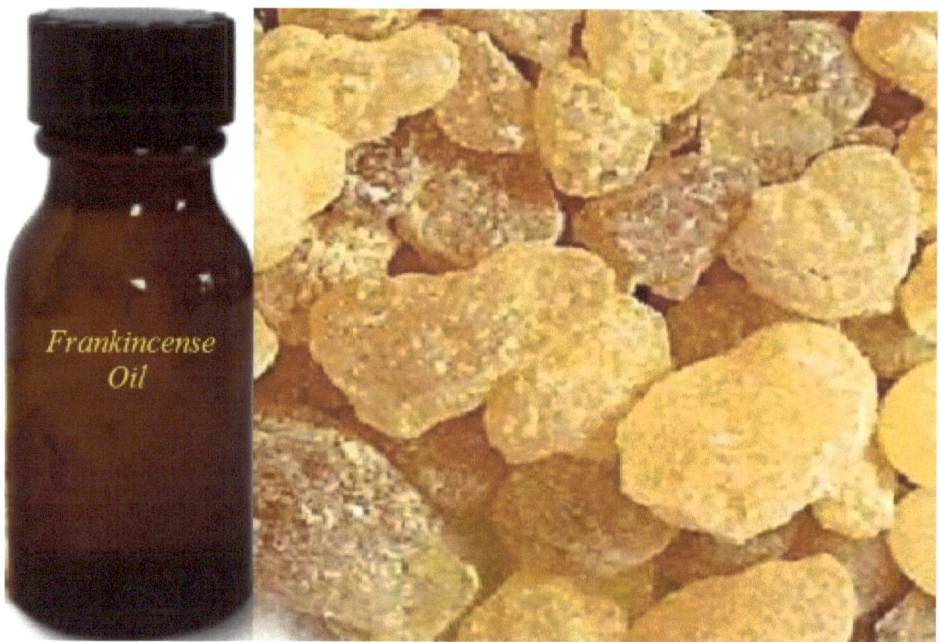

The oil of oils with unmatched healing curative power brought to the king of kings, now available to all of us. In ancient times it was treasured as a medicinal and spiritual tool, treating all health conditions even altering mood and emotion.

There are six types of Frankincense oil made from Boswellia resin. Boswellia carterii from Africa and Boswellia sacra from the Arabian Peninsula are the most common resins used on the market and researched. The other types are worth mentioning, B. frereana, B. serrata, B. thurifera, and B. papyrifera.

Frankincense (Boswellia) is a potent anti-inflammatory agent with no side effects or drug interactions. It blocks the 5-lipoxygenase enzyme which is part of the inflammatory process. This oil treats respiratory, digestive, autoimmune diseases, osteoarthritis, and many other ailments. Used topically it heals wounds, relieves pain, and soothes sore muscles. Taken internally it has been proven to cure cancer, actually stimulates apoptosis (cancer cell death) recognizing healthy cells and not harming them (see references). In Ovarian, breast, pancreatic colon, brain, lung, and bladder cancer Frankincense oil suppressed cancer cell viability. Articles revealing endometriosis patients at high risk for cancer led me to use two drops daily sublingually. When inhaled Frankincense is mood altering and relieves stress and anxiety.

Most important quality for me is the powerful anti-inflammatory action which eliminates pain allows healing from most diseases. Heating it in an oil pot to keeps a pleasant, calm atmosphere in our home.

Frankincense is found many times in the Bible, Leviticus 2: 1-2, 14-16, Leviticus 5: 11, Leviticus 6: 15, Leviticus 24: 7, Numbers 5: 15, 1Chronicles 9: 29, Nehemiah 13: 5, Song of Solomon 3: 6, Son of Solomon 4: 6-16, Mathew 2: 11 (Jesus was born), Revelation 18: 13

Scientific, Medical references are located at the end.

MYRRH

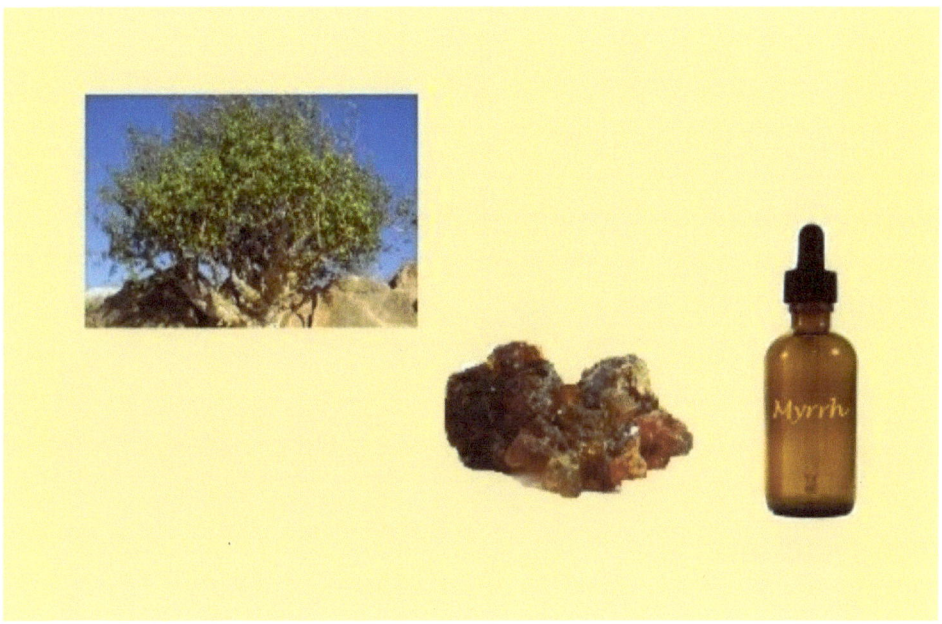

Myrrh (Guggul) sometimes referred to as Oleogum resin from the plant Commiphora myrrha in the Bible is grown in the Middle East. Myrrh was the first oil mentioned in the old testament of the Bible, Genesis 37: 25 and 43: 11 regularly used in ancient times; it was worth more than gold at the time of Jesus birth.

One of the most powerful antioxidants on the market and they lived a long time back then, as in the days of Noah. Its many uses include:

Regulating metabolism

Normalizes T3/ T4 levels in Thyroid function

Weight control

Antioxidant

Anesthetic

Antibacterial

Antifungal

Anti-inflammatory and reduces pain

Wound care

Heals joints and connective tissue

Boost Immunity

Current medical research also shows it suppresses bone tumors, lowers cholesterol, and sesquiterpenes from myrrh inhibit androgen receptors in prostate cancer.

HYSSOP

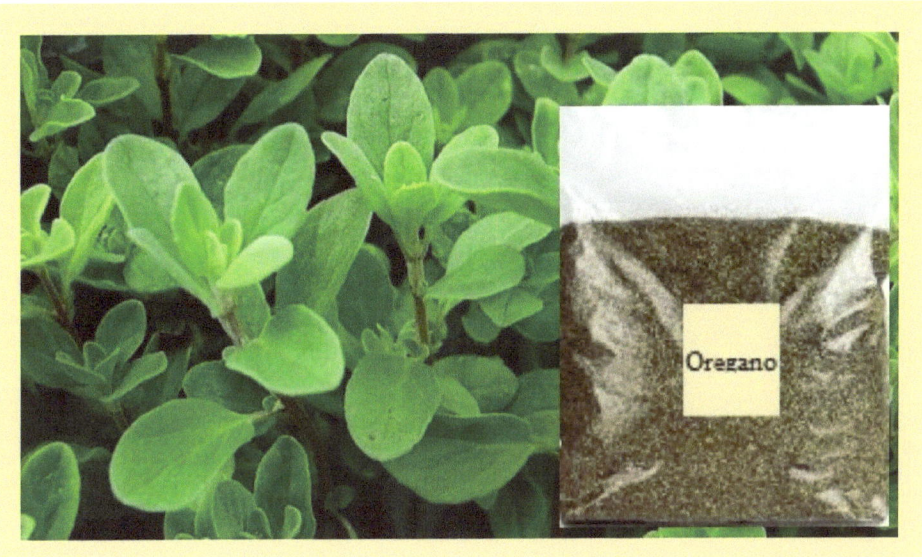

Hyssop is wild Oregano grown in the Mediterranean with Turkey being the largest exporter of Oregano oil. Carvacrol is the main component of biological activity which gives the oil or herb its medicinal value. It is an infection fighter on all levels.

Antifungal

Antibacterial

Antiviral

Antiseptic

Antimicrobial

Anti- parasitic

Anti-inflammatory

Antioxidant

Boost the immune system

Shrinks tumors (so powerful it inhibits HIV replication see references)

I use dried oregano leaves and make a little tea with honey to prevent respiratory infections.

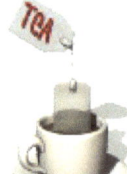

Coconut Oil

Palm Tree Fruit

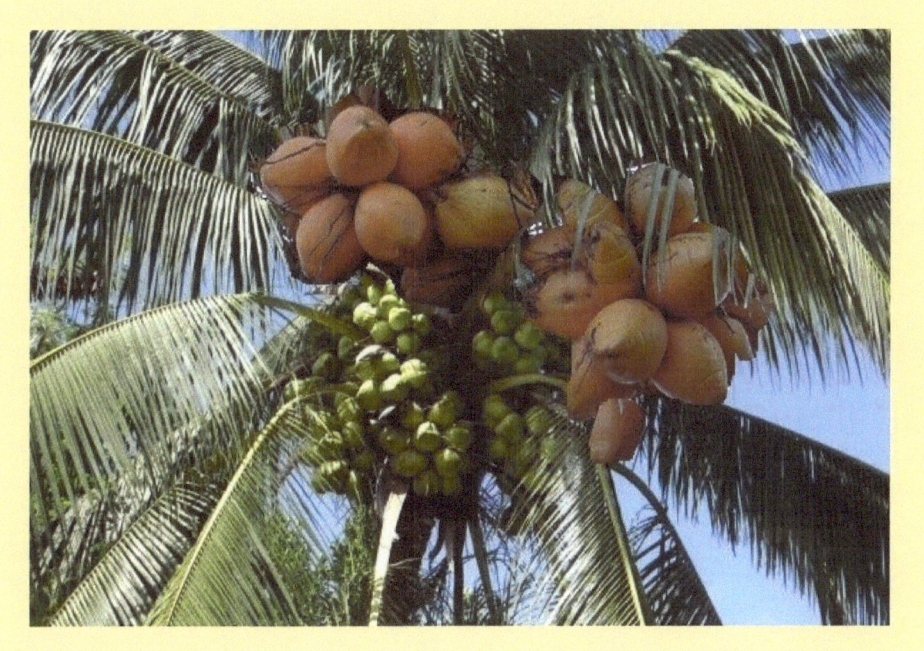

Palm trees are symbolic in my family as a figure of strength; the roots run deep, and the tree can bend to ground in a 150 mph wind and pop back up.

The leaves are huge and provide shade, as well as being a natural air purifier. An unknown miracle the cure for Alzheimer's disease may be hiding in Palm tree fruit, the coconut. An incredible surprise finding while researching my favorite tree has offered unexpected hope to a devastating illness. I am immensely grateful for the work of Dr. Mary Newport, the article titled "What if there was a cure for Alzheimer's disease and no one knew" (2008), started great research for a natural cure.

Palm trees are mentioned several times in the Bible. Psalm 92:12 The righteous shall flourish like the palm-tree: he shall grow like a cedar in Lebanon. Exodus 15: 27- And they came to Elim, where were twelve wells of water, and threescore and ten palm-trees: and they encamped there by the waters. (A beautiful oasis of 70 palm trees described). Other scriptures include Deuteronomy 34: 3; Song of Songs 7: 7-8; and Joel 1: 12.

CHAPTER 5
BREATH OF LIFE

PNEUMA

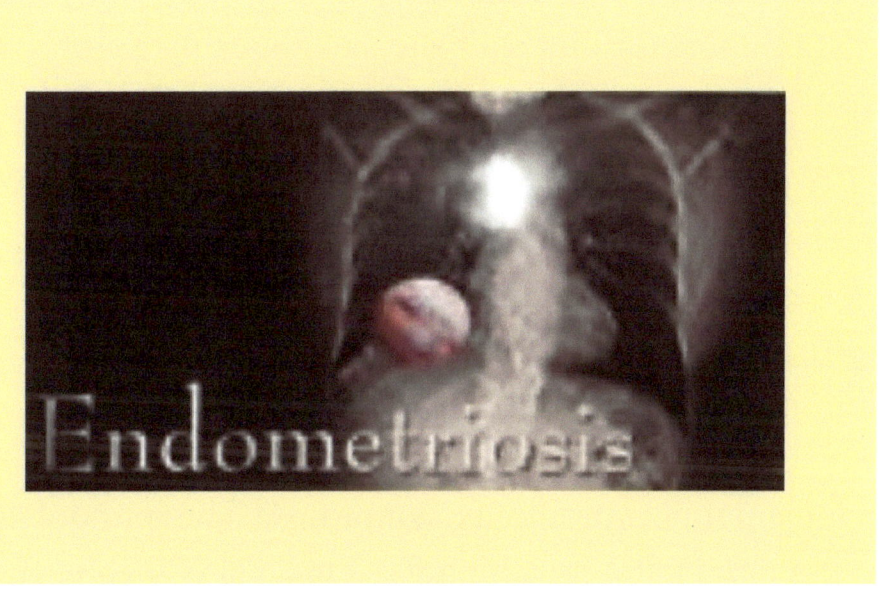

Pneuma defined as the spirit, soul, or creative force of a person. In Greek, it is the word for breath and in religion referred to as wind or spirit, Holy Spirit.

The first thing we see in Genesis is about the spirit. (Genesis 1:2) "And the Spirit of God moved upon the face of the waters." New Testament Pneuma, Luke 24:39 (KJV), Behold my hands and my feet, that it is I: handle me, and see; for a spirit hath not flesh and bones, as ye see me have.

A medical student shared with me, when studying pneumothorax, it felt as if she saw the Holy Spirit inside the lung.

Another fear was not pushing more air to travel to the base of the lung to keep it from collapsing due to atelectasis. I had to find a way to push air on every surface of the lung base. Initially, I used an incentive spirometer, but air filled my stomach also with a bubbling sensation developing as described in catamenial pneumothorax symptoms. The introduction to diaphragmatic breathing gave me a new long term harmonious workable solution. No equipment required this deep breathing technique is accomplished by contracting the diaphragm or belly breathing. I use a 5 10 15 method since 5 is the number of grace.

Slowly breathe in through your nose with your lips pursed tight, hold 10 seconds if possible, blow out through your mouth a minimum of 15 seconds. I blow out until I cough, to make sure I am getting anything that's not supposed to be there out. When you repeat the sequence, a noticeable difference is felt, and I do this at least 2 to 3 times a day or more. You will be amazed at the vibrant awakening energy you feel. Breath is the vital life force that does not tolerate opposition.

CHAPTER 6
MISSION AND PURPOSE REVEALED IN A DREAM

I had a dream. But before I fell asleep, I talked to God about the difficulties of my disease and finances and life in general. I compared myself to the woman with an issue of blood in the Bible who bled for 12 years with no help for her condition but eventually as Jesus passed by, she was able to touch the hem of his garment and faith restored her. All I could think about is if I could just touch, everything would be alright. In my dream that night I was floating in my kitchen close to the ceiling, and could see a man with his back to me.

He had medium brown hair, an off white cotton long robe with a belt around the waist, carrying my limp body with my head hanging back hair almost touching the ground, arms hanging down with hands turned under facing backward. I was completely lifeless and the man was not moving, but the room was very bright, when all of a sudden in my left ear, a stern but kind voice said "Turn your hands up". I sat straight up in bed; fully awake remembering every detail, but what did turn your hands up mean. Maybe my life contributions needed revising, but one afternoon while watching the show I think its supernatural I found the answer. A guy was talking about visitations from Jesus, and he described what Jesus said to him about his hands on the first visit. "Human hands are an extension of heaven they are an extension of my heart. Have an open hand, not a closed fist. Live with an open hand to affirm with, love, touch, bless and heal. Confirmation for me was when he talked about the second visit and the song Jesus sang to him. It was the song I sing to Jesus. Hairs stood up on the back of my neck, with goosebumps from head to toe.

"Have I told you lately that I love you?

Have I told you there is no one else above you?

You fill my heart with gladness, take away all my sadness, ease my   troubles that's what you do,

For the morning sun and all its glory: (that is a morning glory flower on the book cover)

Greet the day with hope and comfort too.

You fill my life laughter; somehow you make it better.

Ease my troubles that's what you do.

There's a love that's divine, and it's yours, and it's mine like the sun. And At the end of the day we should give thanks and pray to the one:

Have I told you lately?

By Rod Stewart

    Jesus had come down for me, and it was time to turn my hand up, and show Gods glory, the cycle of lung bleeding, collapse and fear was over. My mission and purpose was to help others heal.

WOMEN WITH ISSUES OF BLOOD

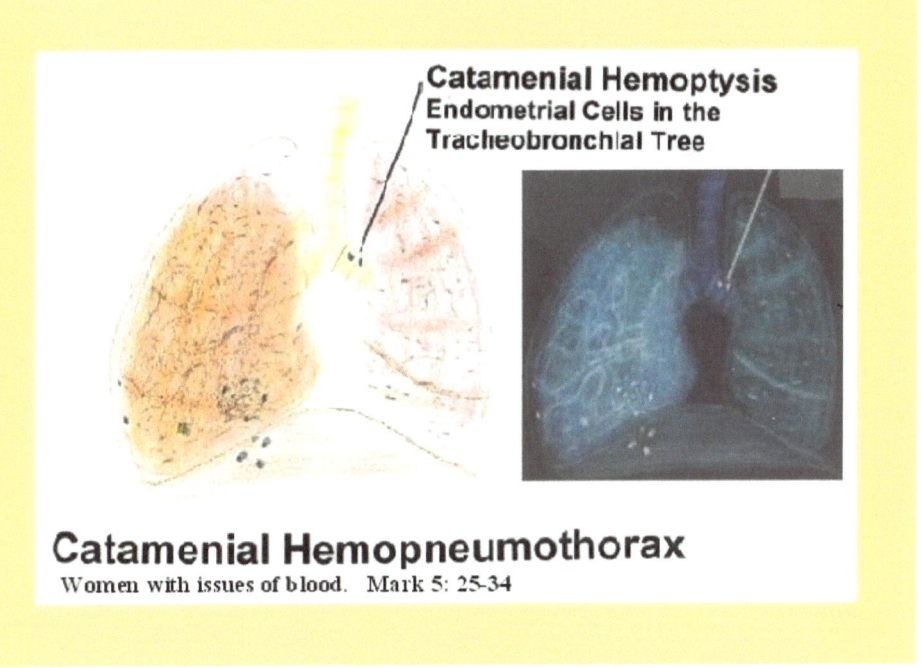

I drew a picture of me touching the hem of his garment inside my collapsed lung and other women and girls with faith seem to show up to be blessed. I call this my Rh negative factor vision.

Starseeds of the world chosen to distribute wisdom and infinite knowledge of the creator, selected to be on earth at this time, I applaud you.

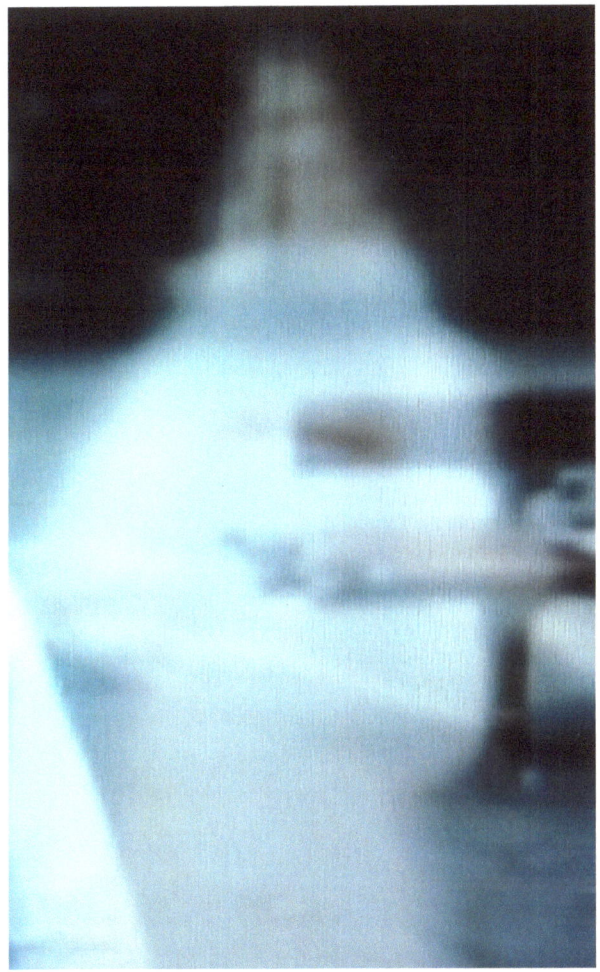

Do not be afraid if you see "Jesus," he is your friend! Jesus, the Son of God, is a healer, and his stories in the Bible are my favorites. Of course, he was much more, but his healing capacity fascinated me.

REFERENCES

Turmeric

Ying Zhang, M.D., Hong Cao, M.D., Zheng Yu, M.D., Hai-Ying Peng, M.D., and Chang-jun Zhang, M.D. **Curcumin inhibits endometriosis endometrial cells by reducing estradiol production**. Iran J Reprod Med. 2013 May; 11(5): 415–422.

Jiang M, Huang O, Zhang X, Xie Z, Shen A, Liu H, Geng M, Shen K **Curcumin induces cell death and restores tamoxifen sensitivity in the antiestrogen-resistant breast cancer cell lines MCF-7/LCC2 and MCF-7/LCC9.** Molecules. 2013 Jan 8;18(1):701-20. doi: 10.3390/molecules18010701.

Ying Zhang M.D., Hong Cao Ph.D., Zheng Yu M.D., Hai-Ying Peng M.D., Chang-jun Zhang M.D. **Nutritional Influences on Estrogen Metabolism**. Iran J Reprod Med Vol. 11. No. 5. pp: 415-422, May 2013.

Frankincense

Rafie Hamidpour, Soheila Hamidpour, Mohsen Hamidpour, Mina Shahlari. Frankincense (乳香 Rǔ Xiāng; Boswellia Species): **From the Selection of Traditional Applications to the Novel Phytotherapy for the Prevention and Treatment of Serious Diseases** J Tradit Complement Med. 2013 Oct-Dec; 3(4): 221–226. doi: 10.4103/2225-4110.119723

Xiao Ni, Mahmoud M Suhail, Qing Yang, Amy Cao,4 Kar-Ming Fung, Russell G Postier, Cole Woolley, Gary Young, Jingzhe Zhang,corresponding author and Hsueh-Kung Lincorresponding. **Frankincense essential oil prepared from hydrodistillation of Boswellia sacra gum resins induces human pancreatic cancer cell death in cultures and in a xenograft murine model.** BMC Complement Altern Med. 2012; 12: 253. Published online 2012 Dec 13. doi: 10.1186/1472-6882-12-253

Mark Barton Frank, Qing Yang, Jeanette Osban, Joseph T Azzarello, Marcia R Saban, Ricardo Saban, Richard A Ashley, Jan C Welter,4 Kar-Ming Fung, and Hsueh-Kung Lin. **Frankincense oil derived from Boswellia carteri induces tumor cell specific cytotoxicity** BMC Complement Altern Med. 2009; 9: 6. Published online 2009 Mar 18. doi: 10.1186/1472-6882-9-6

M. Z. Siddiqui. **Boswellia Serrata, A Potential Antiinflammatory Agent: An Overview**. Indian J Pharm Sci. 2011 May-Jun; 73(3): 255–261. doi: 10.4103/0250-474X.93507

U Siemoneit, A Koeberle, A Rossi, F Dehm, M Verhoff, S Reckel, TJ Maier, J Jauch, H Northoff, F Bernhard, V Doetsch, L Sautebin, and O Werz. **Inhibition of microsomal prostaglandin E2 synthase-1 as a molecular basis for the anti-inflammatory actions of boswellic acids from frankincense** Br J Pharmacol. 2011 Jan; 162(1): 147–162. doi: 10.1111/j.1476-5381.2010.01020.x

Mahmoud M Suhail, Weijuan Wu, Amy Cao, Fadee G Mondalek, Kar-Ming Fung, Pin-Tsen Shih, Yu-Ting Fang, Cole Woolley, Gary Young, Hsueh-Kung Lin. **Boswellia sacra essential oil induces tumor cell-specific apoptosis and suppresses tumor aggressiveness in cultured human breast cancer cells.** BMC Complement Altern Med. 2011; 11: 129. Published online 2011 December 15. doi: 10.1186/1472-6882-11-129 PMCID: PMC3258268

Masanobu Takahashi, Bokyung Sung, Yan Shen, Keun Hur, Alexander Link, C. Richard Boland, Bharat B. Aggarwal, and Ajay Goel. **Boswellic acid exerts antitumor effects in colorectal cancer cells by modulating expression of the let-7 and miR-200 microRNA family.** Carcinogenesis. 2012 Dec; 33(12): 2441–2449. Published online 2012 Sep 16. doi: 10.1093/carcin/bgs286

Myrrh

Shishodia S, Harikumar KB, Dass S, Ramawat KG, Aggarwal BB. **The guggul for chronic diseases: ancient medicine, modern targets**. Anticancer Res. 2008 Nov-Dec;28(6A):3647-64.

Deng R. **Therapeutic effects of guggul and its constituent guggulsterone: cardiovascular benefits**. Cardiovasc Drug Rev. 2007 Winter;25(4):375-90.

Wang XL, Kong F, Shen T, Young CY, Lou HX, Yuan HQ. **Sesquiterpenoids from myrrh inhibit androgen receptor expression and function in human prostate cancer cells.** Acta Pharmacol Sin. 2011 Mar;32(3):338-44. doi: 10.1038/aps.2010.219. PMID: 21372825.

Nomicos EY. **Myrrh: medical marvel or myth of the Magi**? Holist Nurs Pract. 2007 Nov-Dec;21(6):308-23. Review. PMID: 17978635

Dolara P, Corte B, Ghelardini C, Pugliese AM, Cerbai E, Menichetti S, Lo Nostro A. **Local anaesthetic, antibacterial and antifungal properties of sesquiterpenes from myrrh.** Planta Med. 2000 May;66(4):356-8. PMID: 10865454.

Hyssop (Oregano)

Baser KH1. **Biological and pharmacological activities of carvacrol and carvacrol bearing essential oils.** Curr Pharm Des. 2008;14(29):3106-19.

Kreis W1, Kaplan MH, Freeman J, Sun DK, Sarin PS. **Inhibition of HIV replication by Hyssop officinalis extracts.** Antiviral Res. 1990 Dec;14(6):323-37.

Gilling DH1, Kitajima M, Torrey JR, Bright KR. **Antiviral efficacy and mechanisms of action of oregano essential oil and its primary component carvacrol against murine norovirus.** J Appl

Microbiol. 2014 May;116(5):1149-63. doi: 10.1111/jam.12453. Epub 2014 Feb 12

Fan K, Li X, Cao Y, Qi H, Li L, Zhang Q, Sun H. **Carvacrol inhibits proliferation and induces apoptosis in human colon cancer cells.** Anticancer Drugs. 2015 Sep;26(8):813-23. doi: 10.1097/CAD.0000000000000263. PMID: 26214321

Nostro A1, Sudano Roccaro A, Bisignano G, Marino A, Cannatelli MA, Pizzimenti FC, Cioni PL, Procopio F, Blanco AR. **Effects of oregano, carvacrol and thymol on Staphylococcus aureus and Staphylococcus epidermidis biofilms.** J Med Microbiol. 2007 Apr;56(Pt 4):519-23.

Coconut Oil

Mary T. Newport, Theodore B. VanItallie, Yoshihiro Kashiwaya, Michael Todd King, Richard L. Veech. **A new way to produce hyperketonemia: use of ketone ester in a case of Alzheimer's**. Published in final edited form as: Alzheimers Dement. 2015 January; 11(1): 99–103. Published online 2014 October 7. doi: 10.1016/j.jalz.2014.01.006. PMCID: PMC4300286

About the Author

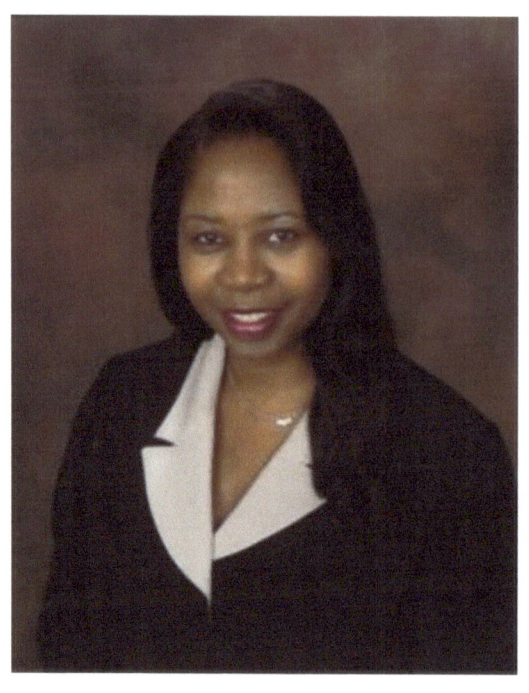

Dr. Glynis D. Wallace, a graduate of Tufts University School of Dental Medicine, former Major in the USAF, internationally known author. Dr. Wallace created the Wikipedia page for Catamenial Pneumothorax in 2006 which stimulated a move to action with undetermined numbers of women being diagnosed globally with Thoracic Endometriosis Syndrome.

OTHER BOOKS BY

DR. GLYNIS D. WALLACE

"Living With Lung and Colon Endometriosis: Catamenial Pneumothorax"

"O RhD Negative (O-) Bloodtype and Catamenial Endometriosis: Catamenial Blood Theories Include Men

ONE LAST THING

If you liked this book, I would be very grateful if you would please leave a short review on Amazon.

www.ingramcontent.com/pod-product-compliance
Lightning Source LLC
Chambersburg PA
CBHW040902180526
45159CB00001B/489